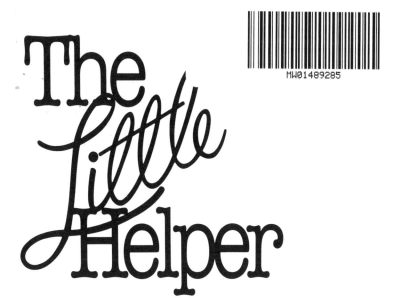

The Little Helper

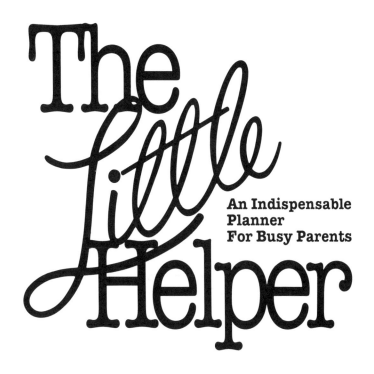

The Little Helper

An Indispensable Planner For Busy Parents

JERRI JOHNSON

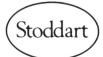

First published in 1988 by
Stoddart Publishing Co. Limited
34 Lesmill Road
Toronto, Canada

Canadian Cataloguing in Publication Data

Johnson, Jerri.
  The little helper

ISBN 0-7737-5122-X

1. First aid in illness and injury - Handbooks, manuals, etc. 2. Pediatric emergencies - Handbooks, manuals, etc. 3. Baby sitters. 4. Planning - Calendars. I. Title.

RJ370.J63 1987
618.92'00252
C87-093902-5

Design: Jerri Johnson
Cover: Brant Cowie/Artplus Limited
Illustrations: Kent Monkman
Printed and bound in Canada

The First Aid material contained in this book has been read and approved by the Canadian Red Cross Society and the Heart and Stroke Foundation of Ontario.

To All Working Parents

This book is dedicated to our children:

(Picture)   (Picture)

Name _____   Name _____
Birthday _____   Birthday _____

(Picture)   (Picture)

Name _____   Name _____
Birthday _____   Birthday _____

Our home address: _____

Contents

Acknowledgements

The author would like to acknowledge The Heart and Stroke Foundation of Ontario, The Canadian Red Cross Society, and the Hospital for Sick Children for their advice and help in collecting the information contained within this book.

Introduction

As a working mother with two small children who are cared for by a sitter, I felt there was a need for a source book where up-to-date information pertaining to my children could be recorded. I found it necessary to have something more concrete and durable than bits and pieces of information scribbled down just before I ran out the door. Therefore, I compiled various subjects which I found essential for the sitter to know in my absence—information I would likely neglect to tell her because of my hectic schedule. Now the sitter will have this information at her fingertips. In the case of an emergency, all the sitter has to do is grab THE LITTLE HELPER and take it to the hospital with her. This book is also helpful in passing daily information back and forth between the sitter and the parents, and for parents to keep their children's activities well in hand.

At the end of the year your manual may be kept as a record of your child's/children's development. It will prove to be invaluable when referring back to a date for important medical information or a significant event such as the day your child said his or her first word. I'm sure you are going to find this manual to be as useful as I have.

Phone List

Emergency _____

Fire _____

Poison Control _____

Taxis _____

_____

_____

	Address	**Phone**

Closest Hospital _____

Police (neighborhood) _____

Neighbor to call in
case of emergency _____

_____

Parent work numbers _____

_____

_____

_____

Name	**Address**	**Phone**

Next of Kin _____

_____

Grandparents _____

_____

_____

Doctors _____

_____

_____

Dentists _____

_____

Bank _____

_____

Closest neighbour's phone number _____

Insurance   Home _____

Life _____

Car _____

Lawyer _____

Accountant _____

Name	**Address**	**Phone**

Schools

1. _____

Principal _____

2. _____

Principal _____

3. _____

Principal _____

4. _____

Principal _____

Teachers _____

_____

_____

_____

Special classes & coaches _____

_____

_____

_____

_____

Name	**Address**	**Phone**

Babysitters:
Emergency sitting services _____

_____

_____

_____

_____

Regular sitters _____

_____

_____

_____

_____

Friends and neighbors _____

_____

_____

_____

_____

_____

_____

Name	Address	Phone
Gas Company		
Furnace Company		
Electric Company		
Water		
Electrician		
Plumber		
Carpenter		
Locksmith		
Vet		
Recreation Centres		
Library		

Medical Charts

Medical Insurance Number _____

Other coverage _____

_____

_____

Dental Insurance _____

When you are going out of town and leaving your child/children in the care of a relative or babysitter for an extended period of time, authorize the caregiver in writing to make decisions concerning medical emergencies. Consult your family doctor for further details concerning this matter.

Notes _____

_____

_____

_____

_____

_____

_____

_____

Name									
Birthdate									
Blood Type									
Shots	Pertussis	Diphtheria	Tetanus	Polio	Oral Polio	Measles	Mumps	Rubella	TB Skin Test
Date									

Name									
Birthdate									
Blood Type									
Shots	Pertussis	Diphtheria	Tetanus	Polio	Oral Polio	Measles	Mumps	Rubella	TB Skin Test
Date									

Name

Birthdate

Blood Type

Shots	Pertussis	Diphtheria	Tetanus	Polio	Oral Polio	Measles	Mumps	Rubella	TB Skin Test
Date									

Name

Birthdate

Blood Type

Shots	Pertussis	Diphtheria	Tetanus	Polio	Oral Polio	Measles	Mumps	Rubella	TB Skin Test
Date									

Allergies

Name _____

_____

_____

_____

Sensitivity to Drugs _____

_____

_____

_____

Name _____

_____

_____

_____

Sensitivity to Drugs _____

_____

_____

_____

Allergies

Name _____

_____

_____

Sensitivity to Drugs _____

_____

_____

_____

Name _____

_____

_____

Sensitivity to Drugs _____

_____

_____

_____

Medical History

Name _____

_____

_____

_____

_____

_____

_____

Name _____

_____

_____

_____

_____

_____

_____

Name _____

_____

_____

_____

_____

_____

_____

Name _____

_____

_____

_____

_____

_____

_____

First Aid

Every home should have a First Aid Kit. The First Aid container should be clean and waterproof.

Every First Aid Kit should contain the following:

A First Aid manual
Triangular bandages (2)
Dressing (Gauze)
Syrup of Ipecac
Adhesive strips

Emergency telephone numbers
Pencil and pad
Blanket
Safety pins
Adhesive tape

Scissors
Tweezers
Change for a phone

Our First Aid Kit is located _____

How to Call Emergency

Don't Panic: Dial Emergency number _____

Speak clearly and give the following information:

1. The location of the emergency including address and names of streets or landmarks.

2. The telephone number from which the call is being made.

3. What happened, i.e. auto accident, poison etc.

4. The number of victims.

5. The condition of victims.

6. The nature of the aid being given.

7. Any other information requested. To ensure that all information requested has been given, the caller should hang up last.

What to do in case of:

Poison

Phone Emergency _____ for an ambulance.

While waiting try to identify the poison, then call the Poison Control Center _____. Staff at the center can begin offering advice after they ask you questions about the type and amount of poison swallowed. They will advise if further action is necessary.

Never induce vomiting unless advised to do so.

Keep the container which held the poison to show the doctor.

Contact parent.

If a chemical poison has gotten into a child's eye or on his skin, wash the area with lukewarm water and call the Poison Control Center.

Burns

1st Degree (minor)
Skin is red, not broken. Immerse the burned area in cool water at once. Contact parent.

2nd Degree (serious)
Skin is blistered. Immerse the burned area in cool water at once. When blisters form, do not puncture them as these are "nature's bandages." If the blisters break, care for the injury as a wound. Take the child to the nearest hospital or to the family doctor for examination. Contact parent.

3rd Degree (critical)
Phone Emergency _____ for ambulance. Apply cool clean water to cool the burned area. Cover the entire burn lightly with a lint-free cloth.

Lie the child down so that his head is lower than the rest of his body until medical help arrives. Contact parent.

Choking

Conscious Child

Ask the child if he is choking. Allow the child to cough up the object by himself if possible. If he needs assistance apply the abdominal thrust technique.

Have someone phone Emergency _____ for an ambulance.

Abdominal thrust technique:

Stand behind the child and place your arms around his midriff. With a clenched fist push in and up on the upper abdomen between the navel and the botton tip of the breastbone. Each thrust should be distinct and delivered with the intent of relieving the airway of the obstruction. Repeat thrusts until either the obstruction is expelled or the child becomes unconscious. See diagram #1.

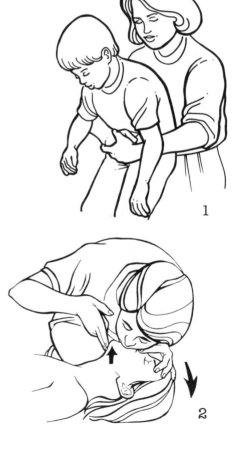

1

Unconscious Child

Step 1. Turn the child on his back, with his face up and his arms by his side. Look into his mouth and remove the obstruction if you can see it. Place your hand on his forehead and tilt his head gently back. With your other hand lift his chin, including the tongue, upward. This is known as the head-tilt/chin-lift manoeuvre and it is important that these two steps be done at the same time. See diagram #2.

2

Pinch his nose tightly with the fingers of the hand that is maintaining the head-tilt. A mouth-to-mouth seal is made. Give two slow breaths. (1 to 1½ seconds per breath) Observe the child's chest rise, and allow the chest to deflate between breaths. See diagram #2.

Step 2. If the child is small (between 1 and 8 years old) lie him on the floor and kneel at his feet, or stand at his feet if he is on a table. A straddle position is recommended for an older child. See diagram #3. Place the heel of one hand against the child's abdomen, in the midline slightly above the navel and well below the tip of the breastbone. Place the second hand directly on top of the first hand. Press into the abdomen with quick upward thrusts. Perform 6 to 10 abdominal thrusts. See diagram #3.

Step 3. Keep the child's face up and open his mouth using the head-tilt/chin-lift manoeuvre. Look into his mouth and remove the obstruction if it is visible.

Repeat steps 1 to 3 until successful.

Contact parent.

3

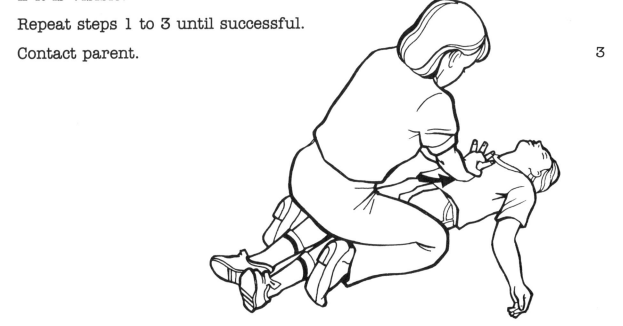

Abdominal Thrust Technique:

Conscious Infant (newborn to 1 year old)

Have someone call Emergency _____ for an ambulance.

Step 1. Straddle infant over your arm or lap keeping his head lower than his trunk. Deliver 4 back blows rapidly and forcefully between the shoulder blades with the heel of the hand.

See diagram #4.

Step 2. Using both your hands to support the infant, turn him on his back. With two fingers, deliver 4 thrusts in the mid-breastbone region. The head is kept lower than the trunk. See diagram #5.

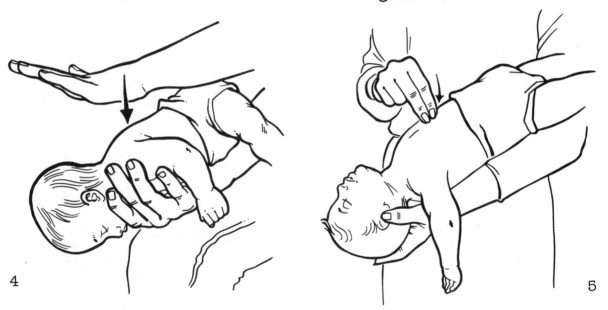

4

5

Alternate the above manoeuvres in rapid sequence. Time is of the essence. If infant becomes unconscious follow the instructions on the next page for unconscious infant.

Unconscious Infant

Step 3. Place your hand on the child's forehead and tilt his head back gently. With your other hand lift his chin including his tongue upward. This is known as the head-tilt/chin-lift manoeuvre and it is important that these two steps be done at the same time. See diagram #6.

Reach with a hooked finger into the infant's throat to remove or dislodge the obstruction if it is visible. <u>Be careful not to drive the object more tightly into the windpipe.</u>

Step 4. Place your mouth on the infant's mouth and nose forming a tight seal. Give small gentle puffs of air. <u>Be careful not to blow too hard and cause damage to the infant's small lungs.</u> Observe the chest rise and allow the chest to deflate between breaths. See diagram #7.
Repeat steps 1 to 4 until successful.

Contact parent.

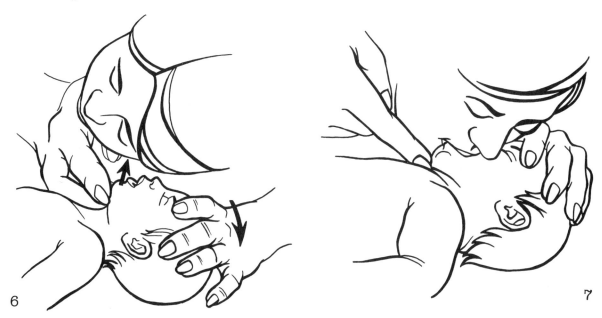

6

7

Mouth-to-Mouth Resuscitation

1. Check to see if child is unconscious. Tap or gently shake the child's shoulder and ask if he is okay as he may be asleep.

2. Phone emergency _____ for an ambulance.

3. Turn the child as a unit on his back, supporting his head and neck. Place him face up and his arms by his side.

4. Make sure the child has an open airway, by using the head-tilt/chin-lift manoeuvre. Place your hand on the child's forehead and tilt his head gently back. With your other hand lift his chin including his tongue upward. It is important that these two steps be done at the same time. See diagram A.

   The head should not be tilted if you suspect a neck injury.

5. Check breathing by looking for movement in the chest and by listening with your ear to the mouth.

6. Look into the child's mouth to see if he is choking. Remove obstruction if visible.

7. Pinch his nose tightly with your fingers of the hand that is maintaining head-tilt.

8. A mouth-to-mouth seal is made. See diagram A.

9. Give two slow breaths. (1 to 1½ seconds per breath)

10. Observe the child's chest rise and allow the chest to deflate between breaths.

11. If the child begins to vomit, roll him over on his side and clear his mouth.

12. Continue mouth-to-mouth resuscitation until successful, or rescue help arrives.

If the victim is an infant, the rescuer's mouth should make a tight seal over the infant's mouth and nose. See diagram B. Since the infant's lungs are smaller, the rescuer should give small puffs of air.

The critical things to remember are:

1. Rescue breaths are the single most important manoeuvre in assisting a non-breathing child.

2. The appropriate volume of air given to the child is that volume which will make the chest rise and fall.

3. By giving breaths slowly, an adequate volume of air will be provided at the lowest possible pressure, so the child's lungs are not damaged.

4. If the air enters freely and the chest rises, the airway is clear. If the chest does not rise the airway is obstructed and the rescuer should apply the abdominal thrust technique to clear the airway.

A
B

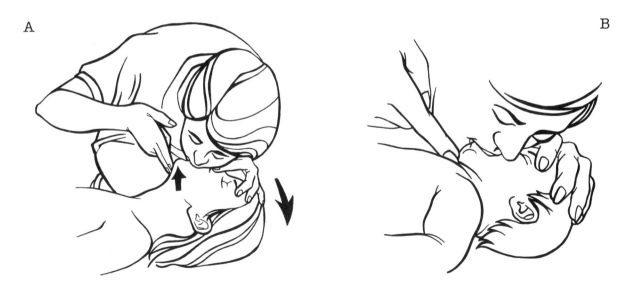

Broken Bones

Phone Emergency _____ for an ambulance to take the child to the nearest hospital. Keep the child warm but do not move the injured limb. Contact parent.

Bumps and Bruises

Comfort the child and apply a cold compress to reduce the swelling. You can make a cold compress by using one of the following methods:

1. Rinse a clean towel or washcloth with cold water and wring out.
2. Wrap an ice cube in a washcloth.
3. Wrap a can of frozen juice in a dry cloth.

Head Injuries

All head injuries are potentially serious and should be reported to the parent. If there are any signs that the child is unwell, notify the family doctor or take the child to the nearest hospital. Apply a cold compress to the injury and watch for any of these signs:

1. Vomiting.
2. Blurred vision or dizziness.
3. Unequal pupil size in the eyes.
4. Bleeding from nose or ears.
5. Severe headache.
6. Drowsiness.
7. Loss of the use of an arm or leg.

Bleeding

Severe: Phone Emergency _____ for an ambulance.

Follow the R.E.D. formula: rest, elevate and direct pressure for all types of bleeding.

Make sure the child is restful, elevate the bleeding area above the level of the heart and place direct pressure on the wound. If there is something protuding from the wound, place pressure on the area around the wound. Contact parent.

Deep cuts: Make a pad out of a clean towel, place on the cut and press firmly on the wound until the bleeding stops. Call family doctor for further advice or take the child to the nearest hospital. Contact parent.

Minor cuts: Clean with soap and water and cover with an adhesive strip.

Nosebleed

Have the child sit on a chair with his head upright. Pinch the nose firmly on either side with thumb and forefinger, where the nasal bone and cartilage meet. Hold firmly for 10 minutes or longer to allow a clot to form. The child's nose should not be blown for 2 hours, or the clot may be dislodged and the bleeding will resume. If the bleeding continues call the family doctor for further advice. Contact parent.

Eye Injury

If dirt, sand, glass or metal is lodged in the surface of the eyeball, instruct the child not to rub the injured eye. Cover both of the child's eyes to reduce eye movement. Tears can wash a foreign body from the eye. The eye may feel sensitive for a short time afterwards, so cover the eye with a light-weight bandage until any discomfort has eased.

Do not attempt to remove a foreign body which has penetrated the surface of the eyeball. Take the child to the nearest hospital immediately. Contact parent.

Ear Injury

If a foreign object is readily seen and easily grasped, it may be gently removed. However, if the object sticks in the ear, do not use an instrument or your fingers to remove it. Take the child to the nearest hospital. Contact parent.

Animal Bites

Wash the bitten area with soap and water. If the skin is broken cover it with a clean cloth. Identify the animal in order that it may be checked for rabies. Contact parent.

Bee and Wasp Stings

Remove the stinger by gently scraping it off the skin. Do not squeeze the stinger by using tweezers or forceps as this could cause the stinger to inject more poison. Apply a cold compress and an application of calamine lotion to the affected area.

Allergic reactions to bee and wasp stings demand immediate attention. The sting could cause immediate swelling of the air passage and the child may need mouth-to-mouth resuscitation.

Phone Emergency _____ for an ambulance.

Follow family doctor's instructions:

_____

_____

_____

_____

_____

pository if instructed by the parent. Keep the child quiet and comfortable. Sit him upright in bed and feed him sips of cool clean liquids such as ice chips, water, carbonated beverages or apple juice.

Contact parent and follow parent's instructions below:

_____

_____

_____

_____

Diarrhea

If the child is vomiting, treat the vomiting first. If the child has diarrhea without vomiting, eliminate solids especially those with roughage such as fruits and vegetables. Eliminate milk as it aggravates diarrhea. Encourage clear liquids such as water, carbonated sodas (allowed to flatten), and iced tea. Watch for blood in stools, high fever and severe or prolonged diarrhea. Contact parent and follow parent's instructions below:

_____

_____

_____

_____

Tooth Injury (baby or permanent)

If the whole tooth including the root is knocked out it may be put back into place.

Clean the tooth by placing it in a bowl of lukewarm water. Do not put it under running water or attempt to wipe it. Carefully replace the tooth in the mouth. It should lock in. Hold the tooth in position while it settles back into place.

Take the child to the dentist or the nearest emergency room immediately. The tooth should be x-rayed to detect any nerve disorder from the accident.

Contact parent.

If the tooth is not holding or you cannot replace it by yourself follow these instructions:

1. Don't attempt to wipe or clean the tooth.

2. Put the tooth in a clean jar of milk or water or wrap it in a damp cloth.

3. Take the child and tooth to his dentist or the nearest emergency room. Time is important. You only have a half an hour in which the tooth can be saved. Contact parent.

Chipped Tooth

If an accident occurs where the child chips his tooth, calm the child and rinse out his mouth with lukewarm water. Contact the parent.

Report a tooth accident to the dentist, even if the tooth isn't chipped especially if you notice the tooth discoloring. The dentist will check for nerve damage. A chipped baby tooth may be filed smooth or bonded for cosmetic reasons. A chipped permanent tooth may be bonded or crowned. Contact your family dentist for further information.

Other Notes

Dayplanner

Week of _____

Monday	Tuesday	Wednesday
8:00	8:00	8:00
9:00	9:00	9:00
10:00	10:00	10:00
11:00	11:00	11:00
12:00	12:00	12:00
1:00	1:00	1:00
2:00	2:00	2:00
3:00	3:00	3:00
4:00	4:00	4:00
5:00	5:00	5:00
6:00	6:00	6:00
7:00	7:00	7:00
8:00	8:00	8:00
Helper's Notes	Helper's Notes	Helper's Notes

	Thursday	Friday	Saturday
8:00		8:00	
9:00		9:00	
10:00		10:00	
11:00		11:00	
12:00		12:00	
1:00		1:00	
2:00		2:00	
3:00		3:00	**Sunday**
4:00		4:00	
5:00		5:00	
6:00		6:00	
7:00		7:00	
8:00		8:00	
Helper's Notes		Helper's Notes	Helper's Notes

Fever

When a child feels cold then hot, this usually signals a fever. If the child appears to be feverish, take his temperature. The human body's normal temperature is 37 degrees C. This may vary 1 degree more or less. If the temperature is over 38 degrees C, notify the parents immediately.

Treatment of the Fever

Keep the child lightly clothed or covered to allow the body heat to escape. Contact parent and follow parent's instructions below:

_____

_____

_____

_____

Common Cold

The symptoms of a child with a cold are sneezing, clear nasal discharge, scratchy sore throat and a fever. Also watch for other symptoms such as dry cough, watery eyes, mild pain in the ears and swollen glands. Contact parent and follow parent's instructions below:

_____

_____

_____

_____

Vomiting

Do not give a child who is vomiting solid foods, milk, or oral aspirin because they can aggravate vomiting. Aspirin may be given by rectal sup-

Week of _____

Monday	Tuesday	Wednesday
8:00	8:00	8:00
9:00	9:00	9:00
10:00	10:00	10:00
11:00	11:00	11:00
12:00	12:00	12:00
1:00	1:00	1:00
2:00	2:00	2:00
3:00	3:00	3:00
4:00	4:00	4:00
5:00	5:00	5:00
6:00	6:00	6:00
7:00	7:00	7:00
8:00	8:00	8:00
Helper's Notes	Helper's Notes	Helper's Notes

Thursday	Friday	Saturday
8:00	8:00	
9:00	9:00	
10:00	10:00	
11:00	11:00	
12:00	12:00	
1:00	1:00	
2:00	2:00	
3:00	3:00	**Sunday**
4:00	4:00	
5:00	5:00	
6:00	6:00	
7:00	7:00	
8:00	8:00	
Helper's Notes	Helper's Notes	Helper's Notes

Week of _____

Monday	Tuesday	Wednesday
8:00	8:00	8:00
9:00	9:00	9:00
10:00	10:00	10:00
11:00	11:00	11:00
12:00	12:00	12:00
1:00	1:00	1:00
2:00	2:00	2:00
3:00	3:00	3:00
4:00	4:00	4:00
5:00	5:00	5:00
6:00	6:00	6:00
7:00	7:00	7:00
8:00	8:00	8:00
Helper's Notes	Helper's Notes	Helper's Notes

Thursday	Friday	Saturday
8:00	8:00	
9:00	9:00	
10:00	10:00	
11:00	11:00	
12:00	12:00	
1:00	1:00	
2:00	2:00	
3:00	3:00	**Sunday**
4:00	4:00	
5:00	5:00	
6:00	6:00	
7:00	7:00	
8:00	8:00	
Helper's Notes	Helper's Notes	Helper's Notes

Week of _____

Monday	Tuesday	Wednesday
8:00	8:00	8:00
9:00	9:00	9:00
10:00	10:00	10:00
11:00	11:00	11:00
12:00	12:00	12:00
1:00	1:00	1:00
2:00	2:00	2:00
3:00	3:00	3:00
4:00	4:00	4:00
5:00	5:00	5:00
6:00	6:00	6:00
7:00	7:00	7:00
8:00	8:00	8:00
Helper's Notes	Helper's Notes	Helper's Notes

Thursday	Friday	Saturday
8:00	8:00	
9:00	9:00	
10:00	10:00	
11:00	11:00	
12:00	12:00	
1:00	1:00	
2:00	2:00	
3:00	3:00	**Sunday**
4:00	4:00	
5:00	5:00	
6:00	6:00	
7:00	7:00	
8:00	8:00	
Helper's Notes	Helper's Notes	Helper's Notes

Week of _____

Monday	Tuesday	Wednesday
8:00	8:00	8:00
9:00	9:00	9:00
10:00	10:00	10:00
11:00	11:00	11:00
12:00	12:00	12:00
1:00	1:00	1:00
2:00	2:00	2:00
3:00	3:00	3:00
4:00	4:00	4:00
5:00	5:00	5:00
6:00	6:00	6:00
7:00	7:00	7:00
8:00	8:00	8:00
Helper's Notes	Helper's Notes	Helper's Notes

Thursday	Friday	Saturday
8:00	8:00	
9:00	9:00	
10:00	10:00	
11:00	11:00	
12:00	12:00	
1:00	1:00	
2:00	2:00	
3:00	3:00	**Sunday**
4:00	4:00	
5:00	5:00	
6:00	6:00	
7:00	7:00	
8:00	8:00	
Helper's Notes	Helper's Notes	Helper's Notes

Week of _____

Monday	Tuesday	Wednesday
8:00	8:00	8:00
9:00	9:00	9:00
10:00	10:00	10:00
11:00	11:00	11:00
12:00	12:00	12:00
1:00	1:00	1:00
2:00	2:00	2:00
3:00	3:00	3:00
4:00	4:00	4:00
5:00	5:00	5:00
6:00	6:00	6:00
7:00	7:00	7:00
8:00	8:00	8:00
Helper's Notes	Helper's Notes	Helper's Notes

Thursday	Friday	Saturday
8:00	8:00	
9:00	9:00	
10:00	10:00	
11:00	11:00	
12:00	12:00	
1:00	1:00	
2:00	2:00	
3:00	3:00	**Sunday**
4:00	4:00	
5:00	5:00	
6:00	6:00	
7:00	7:00	
8:00	8:00	
Helper's Notes	Helper's Notes	Helper's Notes

Week of _____

Monday	Tuesday	Wednesday
8:00	8:00	8:00
9:00	9:00	9:00
10:00	10:00	10:00
11:00	11:00	11:00
12:00	12:00	12:00
1:00	1:00	1:00
2:00	2:00	2:00
3:00	3:00	3:00
4:00	4:00	4:00
5:00	5:00	5:00
6:00	6:00	6:00
7:00	7:00	7:00
8:00	8:00	8:00
Helper's Notes	Helper's Notes	Helper's Notes

Thursday	Friday	Saturday
8:00	8:00	
9:00	9:00	
10:00	10:00	
11:00	11:00	
12:00	12:00	
1:00	1:00	
2:00	2:00	
3:00	3:00	**Sunday**
4:00	4:00	
5:00	5:00	
6:00	6:00	
7:00	7:00	
8:00	8:00	
Helper's Notes	Helper's Notes	Helper's Notes

Week of _____

Monday	Tuesday	Wednesday
8:00	8:00	8:00
9:00	9:00	9:00
10:00	10:00	10:00
11:00	11:00	11:00
12:00	12:00	12:00
1:00	1:00	1:00
2:00	2:00	2:00
3:00	3:00	3:00
4:00	4:00	4:00
5:00	5:00	5:00
6:00	6:00	6:00
7:00	7:00	7:00
8:00	8:00	8:00
Helper's Notes	Helper's Notes	Helper's Notes

Thursday	Friday	Saturday
8:00	8:00	
9:00	9:00	
10:00	10:00	
11:00	11:00	
12:00	12:00	
1:00	1:00	
2:00	2:00	
3:00	3:00	**Sunday**
4:00	4:00	
5:00	5:00	
6:00	6:00	
7:00	7:00	
8:00	8:00	
Helper's Notes	Helper's Notes	Helper's Notes

Week of _____

Monday	Tuesday	Wednesday
8:00	8:00	8:00
9:00	9:00	9:00
10:00	10:00	10:00
11:00	11:00	11:00
12:00	12:00	12:00
1:00	1:00	1:00
2:00	2:00	2:00
3:00	3:00	3:00
4:00	4:00	4:00
5:00	5:00	5:00
6:00	6:00	6:00
7:00	7:00	7:00
8:00	8:00	8:00
Helper's Notes	Helper's Notes	Helper's Notes

Thursday	Friday	Saturday
8:00	8:00	
9:00	9:00	
10:00	10:00	
11:00	11:00	
12:00	12:00	
1:00	1:00	
2:00	2:00	
3:00	3:00	**Sunday**
4:00	4:00	
5:00	5:00	
6:00	6:00	
7:00	7:00	
8:00	8:00	
Helper's Notes	Helper's Notes	Helper's Notes

Week of _____

Monday	Tuesday	Wednesday
8:00	8:00	8:00
9:00	9:00	9:00
10:00	10:00	10:00
11:00	11:00	11:00
12:00	12:00	12:00
1:00	1:00	1:00
2:00	2:00	2:00
3:00	3:00	3:00
4:00	4:00	4:00
5:00	5:00	5:00
6:00	6:00	6:00
7:00	7:00	7:00
8:00	8:00	8:00
Helper's Notes	Helper's Notes	Helper's Notes

Thursday	Friday	Saturday
8:00	8:00	
9:00	9:00	
10:00	10:00	
11:00	11:00	
12:00	12:00	
1:00	1:00	
2:00	2:00	
3:00	3:00	**Sunday**
4:00	4:00	
5:00	5:00	
6:00	6:00	
7:00	7:00	
8:00	8:00	
Helper's Notes	Helper's Notes	Helper's Notes

Week of _____

Monday	Tuesday	Wednesday
8:00	8:00	8:00
9:00	9:00	9:00
10:00	10:00	10:00
11:00	11:00	11:00
12:00	12:00	12:00
1:00	1:00	1:00
2:00	2:00	2:00
3:00	3:00	3:00
4:00	4:00	4:00
5:00	5:00	5:00
6:00	6:00	6:00
7:00	7:00	7:00
8:00	8:00	8:00
Helper's Notes	Helper's Notes	Helper's Notes

Thursday	Friday	Saturday
8:00	8:00	
9:00	9:00	
10:00	10:00	
11:00	11:00	
12:00	12:00	
1:00	1:00	
2:00	2:00	
3:00	3:00	**Sunday**
4:00	4:00	
5:00	5:00	
6:00	6:00	
7:00	7:00	
8:00	8:00	
Helper's Notes	Helper's Notes	Helper's Notes

Week of _____

Monday	Tuesday	Wednesday
8:00	8:00	8:00
9:00	9:00	9:00
10:00	10:00	10:00
11:00	11:00	11:00
12:00	12:00	12:00
1:00	1:00	1:00
2:00	2:00	2:00
3:00	3:00	3:00
4:00	4:00	4:00
5:00	5:00	5:00
6:00	6:00	6:00
7:00	7:00	7:00
8:00	8:00	8:00
Helper's Notes	Helper's Notes	Helper's Notes

Thursday	Friday	Saturday
8:00	8:00	
9:00	9:00	
10:00	10:00	
11:00	11:00	
12:00	12:00	
1:00	1:00	
2:00	2:00	
3:00	3:00	**Sunday**
4:00	4:00	
5:00	5:00	
6:00	6:00	
7:00	7:00	
8:00	8:00	
Helper's Notes	Helper's Notes	Helper's Notes

Week of _____

Monday	Tuesday	Wednesday
8:00	8:00	8:00
9:00	9:00	9:00
10:00	10:00	10:00
11:00	11:00	11:00
12:00	12:00	12:00
1:00	1:00	1:00
2:00	2:00	2:00
3:00	3:00	3:00
4:00	4:00	4:00
5:00	5:00	5:00
6:00	6:00	6:00
7:00	7:00	7:00
8:00	8:00	8:00
Helper's Notes	Helper's Notes	Helper's Notes

Thursday	Friday	Saturday
8:00	8:00	
9:00	9:00	
10:00	10:00	
11:00	11:00	
12:00	12:00	
1:00	1:00	
2:00	2:00	
3:00	3:00	**Sunday**
4:00	4:00	
5:00	5:00	
6:00	6:00	
7:00	7:00	
8:00	8:00	
Helper's Notes	Helper's Notes	Helper's Notes

Week of _____

Monday	Tuesday	Wednesday
8:00	8:00	8:00
9:00	9:00	9:00
10:00	10:00	10:00
11:00	11:00	11:00
12:00	12:00	12:00
1:00	1:00	1:00
2:00	2:00	2:00
3:00	3:00	3:00
4:00	4:00	4:00
5:00	5:00	5:00
6:00	6:00	6:00
7:00	7:00	7:00
8:00	8:00	8:00
Helper's Notes	Helper's Notes	Helper's Notes

Week of _____

Monday	Tuesday	Wednesday
8:00	8:00	8:00
9:00	9:00	9:00
10:00	10:00	10:00
11:00	11:00	11:00
12:00	12:00	12:00
1:00	1:00	1:00
2:00	2:00	2:00
3:00	3:00	3:00
4:00	4:00	4:00
5:00	5:00	5:00
6:00	6:00	6:00
7:00	7:00	7:00
8:00	8:00	8:00
Helper's Notes	Helper's Notes	Helper's Notes

Week of _____

Monday	**Tuesday**	**Wednesday**
8:00	8:00	8:00
9:00	9:00	9:00
10:00	10:00	10:00
11:00	11:00	11:00
12:00	12:00	12:00
1:00	1:00	1:00
2:00	2:00	2:00
3:00	3:00	3:00
4:00	4:00	4:00
5:00	5:00	5:00
6:00	6:00	6:00
7:00	7:00	7:00
8:00	8:00	8:00
Helper's Notes	Helper's Notes	Helper's Notes

Thursday	Friday	Saturday
8:00	8:00	
9:00	9:00	
10:00	10:00	
11:00	11:00	
12:00	12:00	
1:00	1:00	
2:00	2:00	
3:00	3:00	**Sunday**
4:00	4:00	
5:00	5:00	
6:00	6:00	
7:00	7:00	
8:00	8:00	
Helper's Notes	Helper's Notes	Helper's Notes

Week of _____

Monday	Tuesday	Wednesday
8:00	8:00	8:00
9:00	9:00	9:00
10:00	10:00	10:00
11:00	11:00	11:00
12:00	12:00	12:00
1:00	1:00	1:00
2:00	2:00	2:00
3:00	3:00	3:00
4:00	4:00	4:00
5:00	5:00	5:00
6:00	6:00	6:00
7:00	7:00	7:00
8:00	8:00	8:00
Helper's Notes	Helper's Notes	Helper's Notes

## Thursday	## Friday	## Saturday

Thursday	Friday	Saturday
8:00	8:00	
9:00	9:00	
10:00	10:00	
11:00	11:00	
12:00	12:00	
1:00	1:00	
2:00	2:00	
3:00	3:00	**Sunday**
4:00	4:00	
5:00	5:00	
6:00	6:00	
7:00	7:00	
8:00	8:00	
Helper's Notes	Helper's Notes	Helper's Notes

Week of _____

Monday	Tuesday	Wednesday
8:00	8:00	8:00
9:00	9:00	9:00
10:00	10:00	10:00
11:00	11:00	11:00
12:00	12:00	12:00
1:00	1:00	1:00
2:00	2:00	2:00
3:00	3:00	3:00
4:00	4:00	4:00
5:00	5:00	5:00
6:00	6:00	6:00
7:00	7:00	7:00
8:00	8:00	8:00
Helper's Notes	Helper's Notes	Helper's Notes

Thursday	Friday	Saturday
8:00	8:00	
9:00	9:00	
10:00	10:00	
11:00	11:00	
12:00	12:00	
1:00	1:00	
2:00	2:00	
3:00	3:00	**Sunday**
4:00	4:00	
5:00	5:00	
6:00	6:00	
7:00	7:00	
8:00	8:00	
Helper's Notes	Helper's Notes	Helper's Notes

Week of _____

	Monday	**Tuesday**	**Wednesday**
8:00		8:00	8:00
9:00		9:00	9:00
10:00		10:00	10:00
11:00		11:00	11:00
12:00		12:00	12:00
1:00		1:00	1:00
2:00		2:00	2:00
3:00		3:00	3:00
4:00		4:00	4:00
5:00		5:00	5:00
6:00		6:00	6:00
7:00		7:00	7:00
8:00		8:00	8:00
Helper's Notes		Helper's Notes	Helper's Notes

Thursday	Friday	Saturday
8:00	8:00	
9:00	9:00	
10:00	10:00	
11:00	11:00	
12:00	12:00	
1:00	1:00	
2:00	2:00	
3:00	3:00	**Sunday**
4:00	4:00	
5:00	5:00	
6:00	6:00	
7:00	7:00	
8:00	8:00	
Helper's Notes	Helper's Notes	Helper's Notes

Week of _____

Monday	Tuesday	Wednesday
8:00	8:00	8:00
9:00	9:00	9:00
10:00	10:00	10:00
11:00	11:00	11:00
12:00	12:00	12:00
1:00	1:00	1:00
2:00	2:00	2:00
3:00	3:00	3:00
4:00	4:00	4:00
5:00	5:00	5:00
6:00	6:00	6:00
7:00	7:00	7:00
8:00	8:00	8:00
Helper's Notes	Helper's Notes	Helper's Notes

Thursday	Friday	Saturday
8:00	8:00	
9:00	9:00	
10:00	10:00	
11:00	11:00	
12:00	12:00	
1:00	1:00	
2:00	2:00	
3:00	3:00	**Sunday**
4:00	4:00	
5:00	5:00	
6:00	6:00	
7:00	7:00	
8:00	8:00	
Helper's Notes	Helper's Notes	Helper's Notes

Week of _____

Monday	Tuesday	Wednesday
8:00	8:00	8:00
9:00	9:00	9:00
10:00	10:00	10:00
11:00	11:00	11:00
12:00	12:00	12:00
1:00	1:00	1:00
2:00	2:00	2:00
3:00	3:00	3:00
4:00	4:00	4:00
5:00	5:00	5:00
6:00	6:00	6:00
7:00	7:00	7:00
8:00	8:00	8:00
Helper's Notes	Helper's Notes	Helper's Notes

Thursday	Friday	Saturday
8:00	8:00	
9:00	9:00	
10:00	10:00	
11:00	11:00	
12:00	12:00	
1:00	1:00	
2:00	2:00	
3:00	3:00	**Sunday**
4:00	4:00	
5:00	5:00	
6:00	6:00	
7:00	7:00	
8:00	8:00	
Helper's Notes	Helper's Notes	Helper's Notes

Week of _____

Monday	Tuesday	Wednesday
8:00	8:00	8:00
9:00	9:00	9:00
10:00	10:00	10:00
11:00	11:00	11:00
12:00	12:00	12:00
1:00	1:00	1:00
2:00	2:00	2:00
3:00	3:00	3:00
4:00	4:00	4:00
5:00	5:00	5:00
6:00	6:00	6:00
7:00	7:00	7:00
8:00	8:00	8:00
Helper's Notes	Helper's Notes	Helper's Notes

Thursday	Friday	Saturday
8:00	8:00	
9:00	9:00	
10:00	10:00	
11:00	11:00	
12:00	12:00	
1:00	1:00	
2:00	2:00	
3:00	3:00	**Sunday**
4:00	4:00	
5:00	5:00	
6:00	6:00	
7:00	7:00	
8:00	8:00	
Helper's Notes	Helper's Notes	Helper's Notes

Week of _____

Monday	Tuesday	Wednesday
8:00	8:00	8:00
9:00	9:00	9:00
10:00	10:00	10:00
11:00	11:00	11:00
12:00	12:00	12:00
1:00	1:00	1:00
2:00	2:00	2:00
3:00	3:00	3:00
4:00	4:00	4:00
5:00	5:00	5:00
6:00	6:00	6:00
7:00	7:00	7:00
8:00	8:00	8:00
Helper's Notes	Helper's Notes	Helper's Notes

Thursday	Friday	Saturday
8:00	8:00	
9:00	9:00	
10:00	10:00	
11:00	11:00	
12:00	12:00	
1:00	1:00	
2:00	2:00	
3:00	3:00	**Sunday**
4:00	4:00	
5:00	5:00	
6:00	6:00	
7:00	7:00	
8:00	8:00	
Helper's Notes	Helper's Notes	Helper's Notes

Week of _____

Monday	Tuesday	Wednesday
8:00	8:00	8:00
9:00	9:00	9:00
10:00	10:00	10:00
11:00	11:00	11:00
12:00	12:00	12:00
1:00	1:00	1:00
2:00	2:00	2:00
3:00	3:00	3:00
4:00	4:00	4:00
5:00	5:00	5:00
6:00	6:00	6:00
7:00	7:00	7:00
8:00	8:00	8:00
Helper's Notes	Helper's Notes	Helper's Notes

Thursday	Friday	Saturday
8:00	8:00	
9:00	9:00	
10:00	10:00	
11:00	11:00	
12:00	12:00	
1:00	1:00	
2:00	2:00	
3:00	3:00	**Sunday**
4:00	4:00	
5:00	5:00	
6:00	6:00	
7:00	7:00	
8:00	8:00	
Helper's Notes	Helper's Notes	Helper's Notes

Week of _____

Monday	Tuesday	Wednesday
8:00	8:00	8:00
9:00	9:00	9:00
10:00	10:00	10:00
11:00	11:00	11:00
12:00	12:00	12:00
1:00	1:00	1:00
2:00	2:00	2:00
3:00	3:00	3:00
4:00	4:00	4:00
5:00	5:00	5:00
6:00	6:00	6:00
7:00	7:00	7:00
8:00	8:00	8:00
Helper's Notes	Helper's Notes	Helper's Notes

Thursday	Friday	Saturday
8:00	8:00	
9:00	9:00	
10:00	10:00	
11:00	11:00	
12:00	12:00	
1:00	1:00	
2:00	2:00	
3:00	3:00	**Sunday**
4:00	4:00	
5:00	5:00	
6:00	6:00	
7:00	7:00	
8:00	8:00	
Helper's Notes	Helper's Notes	Helper's Notes

Week of _____

Monday	Tuesday	Wednesday
8:00	8:00	8:00
9:00	9:00	9:00
10:00	10:00	10:00
11:00	11:00	11:00
12:00	12:00	12:00
1:00	1:00	1:00
2:00	2:00	2:00
3:00	3:00	3:00
4:00	4:00	4:00
5:00	5:00	5:00
6:00	6:00	6:00
7:00	7:00	7:00
8:00	8:00	8:00
Helper's Notes	Helper's Notes	Helper's Notes

Thursday	Friday	Saturday
8:00	8:00	
9:00	9:00	
10:00	10:00	
11:00	11:00	
12:00	12:00	
1:00	1:00	
2:00	2:00	
3:00	3:00	**Sunday**
4:00	4:00	
5:00	5:00	
6:00	6:00	
7:00	7:00	
8:00	8:00	
Helper's Notes	Helper's Notes	Helper's Notes

Week of _____

Monday	Tuesday	Wednesday
8:00	8:00	8:00
9:00	9:00	9:00
10:00	10:00	10:00
11:00	11:00	11:00
12:00	12:00	12:00
1:00	1:00	1:00
2:00	2:00	2:00
3:00	3:00	3:00
4:00	4:00	4:00
5:00	5:00	5:00
6:00	6:00	6:00
7:00	7:00	7:00
8:00	8:00	8:00
Helper's Notes	Helper's Notes	Helper's Notes

Thursday	Friday	Saturday
8:00	8:00	
9:00	9:00	
10:00	10:00	
11:00	11:00	
12:00	12:00	
1:00	1:00	
2:00	2:00	
3:00	3:00	**Sunday**
4:00	4:00	
5:00	5:00	
6:00	6:00	
7:00	7:00	
8:00	8:00	
Helper's Notes	Helper's Notes	Helper's Notes

Week of _____

	Monday	**Tuesday**	**Wednesday**
8:00		8:00	8:00
9:00		9:00	9:00
10:00		10:00	10:00
11:00		11:00	11:00
12:00		12:00	12:00
1:00		1:00	1:00
2:00		2:00	2:00
3:00		3:00	3:00
4:00		4:00	4:00
5:00		5:00	5:00
6:00		6:00	6:00
7:00		7:00	7:00
8:00		8:00	8:00
Helper's Notes		Helper's Notes	Helper's Notes

Thursday	Friday	Saturday
8:00	8:00	
9:00	9:00	
10:00	10:00	
11:00	11:00	
12:00	12:00	
1:00	1:00	
2:00	2:00	
3:00	3:00	**Sunday**
4:00	4:00	
5:00	5:00	
6:00	6:00	
7:00	7:00	
8:00	8:00	
Helper's Notes	Helper's Notes	Helper's Notes

Week of _____

Monday	Tuesday	Wednesday
8:00	8:00	8:00
9:00	9:00	9:00
10:00	10:00	10:00
11:00	11:00	11:00
12:00	12:00	12:00
1:00	1:00	1:00
2:00	2:00	2:00
3:00	3:00	3:00
4:00	4:00	4:00
5:00	5:00	5:00
6:00	6:00	6:00
7:00	7:00	7:00
8:00	8:00	8:00
Helper's Notes	Helper's Notes	Helper's Notes

Thursday	Friday	Saturday
8:00	8:00	
9:00	9:00	
10:00	10:00	
11:00	11:00	
12:00	12:00	
1:00	1:00	
2:00	2:00	
3:00	3:00	**Sunday**
4:00	4:00	
5:00	5:00	
6:00	6:00	
7:00	7:00	
8:00	8:00	
Helper's Notes	Helper's Notes	Helper's Notes

Week of _____

Monday	Tuesday	Wednesday
8:00	8:00	8:00
9:00	9:00	9:00
10:00	10:00	10:00
11:00	11:00	11:00
12:00	12:00	12:00
1:00	1:00	1:00
2:00	2:00	2:00
3:00	3:00	3:00
4:00	4:00	4:00
5:00	5:00	5:00
6:00	6:00	6:00
7:00	7:00	7:00
8:00	8:00	8:00
Helper's Notes	Helper's Notes	Helper's Notes

Thursday	Friday	Saturday
8:00	8:00	
9:00	9:00	
10:00	10:00	
11:00	11:00	
12:00	12:00	
1:00	1:00	
2:00	2:00	
3:00	3:00	**Sunday**
4:00	4:00	
5:00	5:00	
6:00	6:00	
7:00	7:00	
8:00	8:00	
Helper's Notes	Helper's Notes	Helper's Notes

Week of _____

Monday	Tuesday	Wednesday
8:00	8:00	8:00
9:00	9:00	9:00
10:00	10:00	10:00
11:00	11:00	11:00
12:00	12:00	12:00
1:00	1:00	1:00
2:00	2:00	2:00
3:00	3:00	3:00
4:00	4:00	4:00
5:00	5:00	5:00
6:00	6:00	6:00
7:00	7:00	7:00
8:00	8:00	8:00
Helper's Notes	Helper's Notes	Helper's Notes

Thursday	Friday	Saturday
8:00	8:00	
9:00	9:00	
10:00	10:00	
11:00	11:00	
12:00	12:00	
1:00	1:00	
2:00	2:00	
3:00	3:00	**Sunday**
4:00	4:00	
5:00	5:00	
6:00	6:00	
7:00	7:00	
8:00	8:00	
Helper's Notes	Helper's Notes	Helper's Notes

Week of _____

Monday	Tuesday	Wednesday
8:00	8:00	8:00
9:00	9:00	9:00
10:00	10:00	10:00
11:00	11:00	11:00
12:00	12:00	12:00
1:00	1:00	1:00
2:00	2:00	2:00
3:00	3:00	3:00
4:00	4:00	4:00
5:00	5:00	5:00
6:00	6:00	6:00
7:00	7:00	7:00
8:00	8:00	8:00
Helper's Notes	Helper's Notes	Helper's Notes

Thursday	Friday	Saturday
8:00	8:00	
9:00	9:00	
10:00	10:00	
11:00	11:00	
12:00	12:00	
1:00	1:00	
2:00	2:00	
3:00	3:00	**Sunday**
4:00	4:00	
5:00	5:00	
6:00	6:00	
7:00	7:00	
8:00	8:00	
Helper's Notes	Helper's Notes	Helper's Notes

Week of _____

Monday	Tuesday	Wednesday
8:00	8:00	8:00
9:00	9:00	9:00
10:00	10:00	10:00
11:00	11:00	11:00
12:00	12:00	12:00
1:00	1:00	1:00
2:00	2:00	2:00
3:00	3:00	3:00
4:00	4:00	4:00
5:00	5:00	5:00
6:00	6:00	6:00
7:00	7:00	7:00
8:00	8:00	8:00
Helper's Notes	Helper's Notes	Helper's Notes

Thursday	Friday	Saturday
8:00	8:00	
9:00	9:00	
10:00	10:00	
11:00	11:00	
12:00	12:00	
1:00	1:00	
2:00	2:00	
3:00	3:00	**Sunday**
4:00	4:00	
5:00	5:00	
6:00	6:00	
7:00	7:00	
8:00	8:00	
Helper's Notes	Helper's Notes	Helper's Notes

Week of _____

Monday	Tuesday	Wednesday
8:00	8:00	8:00
9:00	9:00	9:00
10:00	10:00	10:00
11:00	11:00	11:00
12:00	12:00	12:00
1:00	1:00	1:00
2:00	2:00	2:00
3:00	3:00	3:00
4:00	4:00	4:00
5:00	5:00	5:00
6:00	6:00	6:00
7:00	7:00	7:00
8:00	8:00	8:00
Helper's Notes	Helper's Notes	Helper's Notes

Thursday	Friday	Saturday
8:00	8:00	
9:00	9:00	
10:00	10:00	
11:00	11:00	
12:00	12:00	
1:00	1:00	
2:00	2:00	
3:00	3:00	**Sunday**
4:00	4:00	
5:00	5:00	
6:00	6:00	
7:00	7:00	
8:00	8:00	
Helper's Notes	Helper's Notes	Helper's Notes

Week of _____

Monday	Tuesday	Wednesday
8:00	8:00	8:00
9:00	9:00	9:00
10:00	10:00	10:00
11:00	11:00	11:00
12:00	12:00	12:00
1:00	1:00	1:00
2:00	2:00	2:00
3:00	3:00	3:00
4:00	4:00	4:00
5:00	5:00	5:00
6:00	6:00	6:00
7:00	7:00	7:00
8:00	8:00	8:00
Helper's Notes	Helper's Notes	Helper's Notes

Thursday	Friday	Saturday
8:00	8:00	
9:00	9:00	
10:00	10:00	
11:00	11:00	
12:00	12:00	
1:00	1:00	
2:00	2:00	
3:00	3:00	**Sunday**
4:00	4:00	
5:00	5:00	
6:00	6:00	
7:00	7:00	
8:00	8:00	
Helper's Notes	Helper's Notes	Helper's Notes

Week of _____

Monday	Tuesday	Wednesday
8:00	8:00	8:00
9:00	9:00	9:00
10:00	10:00	10:00
11:00	11:00	11:00
12:00	12:00	12:00
1:00	1:00	1:00
2:00	2:00	2:00
3:00	3:00	3:00
4:00	4:00	4:00
5:00	5:00	5:00
6:00	6:00	6:00
7:00	7:00	7:00
8:00	8:00	8:00
Helper's Notes	Helper's Notes	Helper's Notes

Thursday	Friday	Saturday
8:00	8:00	
9:00	9:00	
10:00	10:00	
11:00	11:00	
12:00	12:00	
1:00	1:00	
2:00	2:00	
3:00	3:00	**Sunday**
4:00	4:00	
5:00	5:00	
6:00	6:00	
7:00	7:00	
8:00	8:00	
Helper's Notes	Helper's Notes	Helper's Notes

Week of _____

Monday	Tuesday	Wednesday
8:00	8:00	8:00
9:00	9:00	9:00
10:00	10:00	10:00
11:00	11:00	11:00
12:00	12:00	12:00
1:00	1:00	1:00
2:00	2:00	2:00
3:00	3:00	3:00
4:00	4:00	4:00
5:00	5:00	5:00
6:00	6:00	6:00
7:00	7:00	7:00
8:00	8:00	8:00
Helper's Notes	Helper's Notes	Helper's Notes

Thursday	Friday	Saturday
8:00	8:00	
9:00	9:00	
10:00	10:00	
11:00	11:00	
12:00	12:00	
1:00	1:00	
2:00	2:00	
3:00	3:00	**Sunday**
4:00	4:00	
5:00	5:00	
6:00	6:00	
7:00	7:00	
8:00	8:00	
Helper's Notes	Helper's Notes	Helper's Notes

Week of _____

Monday	Tuesday	Wednesday
8:00	8:00	8:00
9:00	9:00	9:00
10:00	10:00	10:00
11:00	11:00	11:00
12:00	12:00	12:00
1:00	1:00	1:00
2:00	2:00	2:00
3:00	3:00	3:00
4:00	4:00	4:00
5:00	5:00	5:00
6:00	6:00	6:00
7:00	7:00	7:00
8:00	8:00	8:00
Helper's Notes	Helper's Notes	Helper's Notes

Thursday	Friday	Saturday
8:00	8:00	
9:00	9:00	
10:00	10:00	
11:00	11:00	
12:00	12:00	
1:00	1:00	
2:00	2:00	
3:00	3:00	**Sunday**
4:00	4:00	
5:00	5:00	
6:00	6:00	
7:00	7:00	
8:00	8:00	
Helper's Notes	Helper's Notes	Helper's Notes

Week of _____

Monday	Tuesday	Wednesday
8:00	8:00	8:00
9:00	9:00	9:00
10:00	10:00	10:00
11:00	11:00	11:00
12:00	12:00	12:00
1:00	1:00	1:00
2:00	2:00	2:00
3:00	3:00	3:00
4:00	4:00	4:00
5:00	5:00	5:00
6:00	6:00	6:00
7:00	7:00	7:00
8:00	8:00	8:00
Helper's Notes	Helper's Notes	Helper's Notes

Thursday	Friday	Saturday
8:00	8:00	
9:00	9:00	
10:00	10:00	
11:00	11:00	
12:00	12:00	
1:00	1:00	
2:00	2:00	
3:00	3:00	**Sunday**
4:00	4:00	
5:00	5:00	
6:00	6:00	
7:00	7:00	
8:00	8:00	
Helper's Notes	Helper's Notes	Helper's Notes

Week of _____

Monday	Tuesday	Wednesday
8:00	8:00	8:00
9:00	9:00	9:00
10:00	10:00	10:00
11:00	11:00	11:00
12:00	12:00	12:00
1:00	1:00	1:00
2:00	2:00	2:00
3:00	3:00	3:00
4:00	4:00	4:00
5:00	5:00	5:00
6:00	6:00	6:00
7:00	7:00	7:00
8:00	8:00	8:00
Helper's Notes	Helper's Notes	Helper's Notes

Thursday	Friday	Saturday
8:00	8:00	
9:00	9:00	
10:00	10:00	
11:00	11:00	
12:00	12:00	
1:00	1:00	
2:00	2:00	
3:00	3:00	**Sunday**
4:00	4:00	
5:00	5:00	
6:00	6:00	
7:00	7:00	
8:00	8:00	
Helper's Notes	Helper's Notes	Helper's Notes

Week of _____

Monday	Tuesday	Wednesday
8:00	8:00	8:00
9:00	9:00	9:00
10:00	10:00	10:00
11:00	11:00	11:00
12:00	12:00	12:00
1:00	1:00	1:00
2:00	2:00	2:00
3:00	3:00	3:00
4:00	4:00	4:00
5:00	5:00	5:00
6:00	6:00	6:00
7:00	7:00	7:00
8:00	8:00	8:00
Helper's Notes	Helper's Notes	Helper's Notes

Thursday	Friday	Saturday
8:00	8:00	
9:00	9:00	
10:00	10:00	
11:00	11:00	
12:00	12:00	
1:00	1:00	
2:00	2:00	
3:00	3:00	**Sunday**
4:00	4:00	
5:00	5:00	
6:00	6:00	
7:00	7:00	
8:00	8:00	
Helper's Notes	Helper's Notes	Helper's Notes

Week of _____

Monday	Tuesday	Wednesday
8:00	8:00	8:00
9:00	9:00	9:00
10:00	10:00	10:00
11:00	11:00	11:00
12:00	12:00	12:00
1:00	1:00	1:00
2:00	2:00	2:00
3:00	3:00	3:00
4:00	4:00	4:00
5:00	5:00	5:00
6:00	6:00	6:00
7:00	7:00	7:00
8:00	8:00	8:00
Helper's Notes	Helper's Notes	Helper's Notes

Thursday	Friday	Saturday
8:00	8:00	
9:00	9:00	
10:00	10:00	
11:00	11:00	
12:00	12:00	
1:00	1:00	
2:00	2:00	
3:00	3:00	**Sunday**
4:00	4:00	
5:00	5:00	
6:00	6:00	
7:00	7:00	
8:00	8:00	
Helper's Notes	Helper's Notes	Helper's Notes

Week of _____

Monday	Tuesday	Wednesday
8:00	8:00	8:00
9:00	9:00	9:00
10:00	10:00	10:00
11:00	11:00	11:00
12:00	12:00	12:00
1:00	1:00	1:00
2:00	2:00	2:00
3:00	3:00	3:00
4:00	4:00	4:00
5:00	5:00	5:00
6:00	6:00	6:00
7:00	7:00	7:00
8:00	8:00	8:00
Helper's Notes	Helper's Notes	Helper's Notes

Thursday	Friday	Saturday
8:00	8:00	
9:00	9:00	
10:00	10:00	
11:00	11:00	
12:00	12:00	
1:00	1:00	
2:00	2:00	
3:00	3:00	**Sunday**
4:00	4:00	
5:00	5:00	
6:00	6:00	
7:00	7:00	
8:00	8:00	
Helper's Notes	Helper's Notes	Helper's Notes

Week of _____

Monday	Tuesday	Wednesday
8:00	8:00	8:00
9:00	9:00	9:00
10:00	10:00	10:00
11:00	11:00	11:00
12:00	12:00	12:00
1:00	1:00	1:00
2:00	2:00	2:00
3:00	3:00	3:00
4:00	4:00	4:00
5:00	5:00	5:00
6:00	6:00	6:00
7:00	7:00	7:00
8:00	8:00	8:00
Helper's Notes	Helper's Notes	Helper's Notes

Thursday	Friday	Saturday
8:00	8:00	
9:00	9:00	
10:00	10:00	
11:00	11:00	
12:00	12:00	
1:00	1:00	
2:00	2:00	
3:00	3:00	**Sunday**
4:00	4:00	
5:00	5:00	
6:00	6:00	
7:00	7:00	
8:00	8:00	
Helper's Notes	Helper's Notes	Helper's Notes

Week of _____

Monday	Tuesday	Wednesday
8:00	8:00	8:00
9:00	9:00	9:00
10:00	10:00	10:00
11:00	11:00	11:00
12:00	12:00	12:00
1:00	1:00	1:00
2:00	2:00	2:00
3:00	3:00	3:00
4:00	4:00	4:00
5:00	5:00	5:00
6:00	6:00	6:00
7:00	7:00	7:00
8:00	8:00	8:00
Helper's Notes	Helper's Notes	Helper's Notes

Thursday	Friday	Saturday
8:00	8:00	
9:00	9:00	
10:00	10:00	
11:00	11:00	
12:00	12:00	
1:00	1:00	
2:00	2:00	
3:00	3:00	**Sunday**
4:00	4:00	
5:00	5:00	
6:00	6:00	
7:00	7:00	
8:00	8:00	
Helper's Notes	Helper's Notes	Helper's Notes

Week of _____

Monday	Tuesday	Wednesday
8:00	8:00	8:00
9:00	9:00	9:00
10:00	10:00	10:00
11:00	11:00	11:00
12:00	12:00	12:00
1:00	1:00	1:00
2:00	2:00	2:00
3:00	3:00	3:00
4:00	4:00	4:00
5:00	5:00	5:00
6:00	6:00	6:00
7:00	7:00	7:00
8:00	8:00	8:00
Helper's Notes	Helper's Notes	Helper's Notes

Thursday	Friday	Saturday
8:00	8:00	
9:00	9:00	
10:00	10:00	
11:00	11:00	
12:00	12:00	
1:00	1:00	
2:00	2:00	
3:00	3:00	**Sunday**
4:00	4:00	
5:00	5:00	
6:00	6:00	
7:00	7:00	
8:00	8:00	
Helper's Notes	Helper's Notes	Helper's Notes

Week of _____

Monday	Tuesday	Wednesday
8:00	8:00	8:00
9:00	9:00	9:00
10:00	10:00	10:00
11:00	11:00	11:00
12:00	12:00	12:00
1:00	1:00	1:00
2:00	2:00	2:00
3:00	3:00	3:00
4:00	4:00	4:00
5:00	5:00	5:00
6:00	6:00	6:00
7:00	7:00	7:00
8:00	8:00	8:00
Helper's Notes	Helper's Notes	Helper's Notes

Thursday	Friday	Saturday
8:00	8:00	
9:00	9:00	
10:00	10:00	
11:00	11:00	
12:00	12:00	
1:00	1:00	
2:00	2:00	
3:00	3:00	**Sunday**
4:00	4:00	
5:00	5:00	
6:00	6:00	
7:00	7:00	
8:00	8:00	
Helper's Notes	Helper's Notes	Helper's Notes

Week of _____

Monday	Tuesday	Wednesday
8:00	8:00	8:00
9:00	9:00	9:00
10:00	10:00	10:00
11:00	11:00	11:00
12:00	12:00	12:00
1:00	1:00	1:00
2:00	2:00	2:00
3:00	3:00	3:00
4:00	4:00	4:00
5:00	5:00	5:00
6:00	6:00	6:00
7:00	7:00	7:00
8:00	8:00	8:00
Helper's Notes	Helper's Notes	Helper's Notes

Thursday	Friday	Saturday
8:00	8:00	
9:00	9:00	
10:00	10:00	
11:00	11:00	
12:00	12:00	
1:00	1:00	
2:00	2:00	
3:00	3:00	**Sunday**
4:00	4:00	
5:00	5:00	
6:00	6:00	
7:00	7:00	
8:00	8:00	
Helper's Notes	Helper's Notes	Helper's Notes

Week of _____

Monday	Tuesday	Wednesday
8:00	8:00	8:00
9:00	9:00	9:00
10:00	10:00	10:00
11:00	11:00	11:00
12:00	12:00	12:00
1:00	1:00	1:00
2:00	2:00	2:00
3:00	3:00	3:00
4:00	4:00	4:00
5:00	5:00	5:00
6:00	6:00	6:00
7:00	7:00	7:00
8:00	8:00	8:00
Helper's Notes	Helper's Notes	Helper's Notes

Thursday	Friday	Saturday
8:00	8:00	
9:00	9:00	
10:00	10:00	
11:00	11:00	
12:00	12:00	
1:00	1:00	
2:00	2:00	
3:00	3:00	**Sunday**
4:00	4:00	
5:00	5:00	
6:00	6:00	
7:00	7:00	
8:00	8:00	
Helper's Notes	Helper's Notes	Helper's Notes

Week of _____

Monday	Tuesday	Wednesday
8:00	8:00	8:00
9:00	9:00	9:00
10:00	10:00	10:00
11:00	11:00	11:00
12:00	12:00	12:00
1:00	1:00	1:00
2:00	2:00	2:00
3:00	3:00	3:00
4:00	4:00	4:00
5:00	5:00	5:00
6:00	6:00	6:00
7:00	7:00	7:00
8:00	8:00	8:00
Helper's Notes	Helper's Notes	Helper's Notes

Thursday	Friday	Saturday
8:00	8:00	
9:00	9:00	
10:00	10:00	
11:00	11:00	
12:00	12:00	
1:00	1:00	
2:00	2:00	
3:00	3:00	**Sunday**
4:00	4:00	
5:00	5:00	
6:00	6:00	
7:00	7:00	
8:00	8:00	
Helper's Notes	Helper's Notes	Helper's Notes

Week of _____

Monday	Tuesday	Wednesday
8:00	8:00	8:00
9:00	9:00	9:00
10:00	10:00	10:00
11:00	11:00	11:00
12:00	12:00	12:00
1:00	1:00	1:00
2:00	2:00	2:00
3:00	3:00	3:00
4:00	4:00	4:00
5:00	5:00	5:00
6:00	6:00	6:00
7:00	7:00	7:00
8:00	8:00	8:00
Helper's Notes	Helper's Notes	Helper's Notes

Thursday	Friday	Saturday
8:00	8:00	
9:00	9:00	
10:00	10:00	
11:00	11:00	
12:00	12:00	
1:00	1:00	
2:00	2:00	
3:00	3:00	**Sunday**
4:00	4:00	
5:00	5:00	
6:00	6:00	
7:00	7:00	
8:00	8:00	
Helper's Notes	Helper's Notes	Helper's Notes

Week of _____

Monday	Tuesday	Wednesday
8:00	8:00	8:00
9:00	9:00	9:00
10:00	10:00	10:00
11:00	11:00	11:00
12:00	12:00	12:00
1:00	1:00	1:00
2:00	2:00	2:00
3:00	3:00	3:00
4:00	4:00	4:00
5:00	5:00	5:00
6:00	6:00	6:00
7:00	7:00	7:00
8:00	8:00	8:00
Helper's Notes	Helper's Notes	Helper's Notes

Thursday	Friday	Saturday
8:00	8:00	
9:00	9:00	
10:00	10:00	
11:00	11:00	
12:00	12:00	
1:00	1:00	
2:00	2:00	
3:00	3:00	**Sunday**
4:00	4:00	
5:00	5:00	
6:00	6:00	
7:00	7:00	
8:00	8:00	
Helper's Notes	Helper's Notes	Helper's Notes

Week of _____

Monday	Tuesday	Wednesday
8:00	8:00	8:00
9:00	9:00	9:00
10:00	10:00	10:00
11:00	11:00	11:00
12:00	12:00	12:00
1:00	1:00	1:00
2:00	2:00	2:00
3:00	3:00	3:00
4:00	4:00	4:00
5:00	5:00	5:00
6:00	6:00	6:00
7:00	7:00	7:00
8:00	8:00	8:00
Helper's Notes	Helper's Notes	Helper's Notes

Thursday	Friday	Saturday
8:00	8:00	
9:00	9:00	
10:00	10:00	
11:00	11:00	
12:00	12:00	
1:00	1:00	
2:00	2:00	
3:00	3:00	**Sunday**
4:00	4:00	
5:00	5:00	
6:00	6:00	
7:00	7:00	
8:00	8:00	
Helper's Notes	Helper's Notes	Helper's Notes

Week of _____

Monday	Tuesday	Wednesday
8:00	8:00	8:00
9:00	9:00	9:00
10:00	10:00	10:00
11:00	11:00	11:00
12:00	12:00	12:00
1:00	1:00	1:00
2:00	2:00	2:00
3:00	3:00	3:00
4:00	4:00	4:00
5:00	5:00	5:00
6:00	6:00	6:00
7:00	7:00	7:00
8:00	8:00	8:00
Helper's Notes	Helper's Notes	Helper's Notes

1988

JANUARY
S	M	T	W	T	F	S
					1	2
3	4	5	6	7	8	9
10	11	12	13	14	15	16
17	18	19	20	21	22	23
24	25	26	27	28	29	30
31						

MAY
S	M	T	W	T	F	S
1	2	3	4	5	6	7
8	9	10	11	12	13	14
15	16	17	18	19	20	21
22	23	24	25	26	27	28
29	30	31				

SEPTEMBER
S	M	T	W	T	F	S
				1	2	3
4	5	6	7	8	9	10
11	12	13	14	15	16	17
18	19	20	21	22	23	24
25	26	27	28	29	30	

FEBRUARY
S	M	T	W	T	F	S
	1	2	3	4	5	6
7	8	9	10	11	12	13
14	15	16	17	18	19	20
21	22	23	24	25	26	27
28	29					

JUNE
S	M	T	W	T	F	S
			1	2	3	4
5	6	7	8	9	10	11
12	13	14	15	16	17	18
19	20	21	22	23	24	25
26	27	28	29	30		

OCTOBER
S	M	T	W	T	F	S
						1
2	3	4	5	6	7	8
9	10	11	12	13	14	15
16	17	18	19	20	21	22
23	24	25	26	27	28	29
30	31					

MARCH
S	M	T	W	T	F	S
		1	2	3	4	5
6	7	8	9	10	11	12
13	14	15	16	17	18	19
20	21	22	23	24	25	26
27	28	29	30	31		

JULY
S	M	T	W	T	F	S
					1	2
3	4	5	6	7	8	9
10	11	12	13	14	15	16
17	18	19	20	21	22	23
24	25	26	27	28	29	30
31						

NOVEMBER
S	M	T	W	T	F	S
		1	2	3	4	5
6	7	8	9	10	11	12
13	14	15	16	17	18	19
20	21	22	23	24	25	26
27	28	29	30			

APRIL
S	M	T	W	T	F	S
					1	2
3	4	5	6	7	8	9
10	11	12	13	14	15	16
17	18	19	20	21	22	23
24	25	26	27	28	29	30

AUGUST
S	M	T	W	T	F	S
	1	2	3	4	5	6
7	8	9	10	11	12	13
14	15	16	17	18	19	20
21	22	23	24	25	26	27
28	29	30	31			

DECEMBER
S	M	T	W	T	F	S
				1	2	3
4	5	6	7	8	9	10
11	12	13	14	15	16	17
18	19	20	21	22	23	24
25	26	27	28	29	30	31

1989

JANUARY
S	M	T	W	T	F	S
1	2	3	4	5	6	7
8	9	10	11	12	13	14
15	16	17	18	19	20	21
22	23	24	25	26	27	28
29	30	31				

MAY
S	M	T	W	T	F	S
	1	2	3	4	5	6
7	8	9	10	11	12	13
14	15	16	17	18	19	20
21	22	23	24	25	26	27
28	29	30	31			

SEPTEMBER
S	M	T	W	T	F	S
					1	2
3	4	5	6	7	8	9
10	11	12	13	14	15	16
17	18	19	20	21	22	23
24	25	26	27	28	29	30

FEBRUARY
S	M	T	W	T	F	S
			1	2	3	4
5	6	7	8	9	10	11
12	13	14	15	16	17	18
19	20	21	22	23	24	25
26	27	28				

JUNE
S	M	T	W	T	F	S
				1	2	3
4	5	6	7	8	9	10
11	12	13	14	15	16	17
18	19	20	21	22	23	24
25	26	27	28	29	30	

OCTOBER
S	M	T	W	T	F	S
1	2	3	4	5	6	7
8	9	10	11	12	13	14
15	16	17	18	19	20	21
22	23	24	25	26	27	28
29	30	31				

MARCH
S	M	T	W	T	F	S
			1	2	3	4
5	6	7	8	9	10	11
12	13	14	15	16	17	18
19	20	21	22	23	24	25
26	27	28	29	30	31	

JULY
S	M	T	W	T	F	S
						1
2	3	4	5	6	7	8
9	10	11	12	13	14	15
16	17	18	19	20	21	22
23	24	25	26	27	28	29
30	31					

NOVEMBER
S	M	T	W	T	F	S
			1	2	3	4
5	6	7	8	9	10	11
12	13	14	15	16	17	18
19	20	21	22	23	24	25
26	27	28	29	30		

APRIL
S	M	T	W	T	F	S
						1
2	3	4	5	6	7	8
9	10	11	12	13	14	15
16	17	18	19	20	21	22
23	24	25	26	27	28	29
30						

AUGUST
S	M	T	W	T	F	S
		1	2	3	4	5
6	7	8	9	10	11	12
13	14	15	16	17	18	19
20	21	22	23	24	25	26
27	28	29	30	31		

DECEMBER
S	M	T	W	T	F	S
					1	2
3	4	5	6	7	8	9
10	11	12	13	14	15	16
17	18	19	20	21	22	23
24	25	26	27	28	29	30
31						

1990

JANUARY
S	M	T	W	T	F	S
	1	2	3	4	5	
6	7	8	9	10	11	12
13	14	15	16	17	18	19
20	21	22	23	24	25	26
27	28	29	30	31		

FEBRUARY
S	M	T	W	T	F	S
				1	2	
3	4	5	6	7	8	9
10	11	12	13	14	15	16
17	18	19	20	21	22	23
24	25	26	27	28		

MARCH
S	M	T	W	T	F	S
				1	2	
3	4	5	6	7	8	9
10	11	12	13	14	15	16
17	18	19	20	21	22	23
24	25	26	27	28	29	30
31						

APRIL
S	M	T	W	T	F	S
1	2	3	4	5	6	
7	8	9	10	11	12	13
14	15	16	17	18	19	20
21	22	23	24	25	26	27
28	29	30				

MAY
S	M	T	W	T	F	S
		1	2	3	4	
5	6	7	8	9	10	11
12	13	14	15	16	17	18
19	20	21	22	23	24	25
26	27	28	29	30	31	

JUNE
S	M	T	W	T	F	S
					1	
2	3	4	5	6	7	8
9	10	11	12	13	14	15
16	17	18	19	20	21	22
23	24	25	26	27	28	29
30						

JULY
S	M	T	W	T	F	S
1	2	3	4	5	6	
7	8	9	10	11	12	13
14	15	16	17	18	19	20
21	22	23	24	25	26	27
28	29	30	31			

AUGUST
S	M	T	W	T	F	S
			1	2	3	
4	5	6	7	8	9	10
11	12	13	14	15	16	17
18	19	20	21	22	23	24
25	26	27	28	29	30	31

SEPTEMBER
S	M	T	W	T	F	S
1	2	3	4	5	6	7
8	9	10	11	12	13	14
15	16	17	18	19	20	21
22	23	24	25	26	27	28
29	30					

OCTOBER
S	M	T	W	T	F	S
	1	2	3	4	5	
6	7	8	9	10	11	12
13	14	15	16	17	18	19
20	21	22	23	24	25	26
27	28	29	30	31		

NOVEMBER
S	M	T	W	T	F	S
				1	2	
3	4	5	6	7	8	9
10	11	12	13	14	15	16
17	18	19	20	21	22	23
24	25	26	27	28	29	30

DECEMBER
S	M	T	W	T	F	S
1	2	3	4	5	6	7
8	9	10	11	12	13	14
15	16	17	18	19	20	21
22	23	24	25	26	27	28
29	30	31				

1991

JANUARY
S	M	T	W	T	F	S
	1	2	3	4	5	6
7	8	9	10	11	12	13
14	15	16	17	18	19	20
21	22	23	24	25	26	27
28	29	30	31			

FEBRUARY
S	M	T	W	T	F	S
				1	2	3
4	5	6	7	8	9	10
11	12	13	14	15	16	17
18	19	20	21	22	23	24
25	26	27	28			

MARCH
S	M	T	W	T	F	S
				1	2	3
4	5	6	7	8	9	10
11	12	13	14	15	16	17
18	19	20	21	22	23	24
25	26	27	28	29	30	31

APRIL
S	M	T	W	T	F	S
1	2	3	4	5	6	7
8	9	10	11	12	13	14
15	16	17	18	19	20	21
22	23	24	25	26	27	28
29	30					

MAY
S	M	T	W	T	F	S
		1	2	3	4	
5	6	7	8	9	10	11
12	13	14	15	16	17	18
19	20	21	22	23	24	25
26	27	28	29	30	31	

JUNE
S	M	T	W	T	F	S
					1	
2	3	4	5	6	7	8
9	10	11	12	13	14	15
16	17	18	19	20	21	22
23	24	25	26	27	28	29
30						

JULY
S	M	T	W	T	F	S
	1	2	3	4	5	6
7	8	9	10	11	12	13
14	15	16	17	18	19	20
21	22	23	24	25	26	27
28	29	30	31			

AUGUST
S	M	T	W	T	F	S
				1	2	3
4	5	6	7	8	9	10
11	12	13	14	15	16	17
18	19	20	21	22	23	24
25	26	27	28	29	30	31

SEPTEMBER
S	M	T	W	T	F	S
1						
2	3	4	5	6	7	8
9	10	11	12	13	14	15
16	17	18	19	20	21	22
23	24	25	26	27	28	29
30						

OCTOBER
S	M	T	W	T	F	S
	1	2	3	4	5	6
7	8	9	10	11	12	13
14	15	16	17	18	19	20
21	22	23	24	25	26	27
28	29	30	31			

NOVEMBER
S	M	T	W	T	F	S
				1	2	3
4	5	6	7	8	9	10
11	12	13	14	15	16	17
18	19	20	21	22	23	24
25	26	27	28	29	30	

DECEMBER
S	M	T	W	T	F	S
1						
2	3	4	5	6	7	8
9	10	11	12	13	14	15
16	17	18	19	20	21	22
23	24	25	26	27	28	29
30	31					